How I Beat Crohn's

Through Diet Alone

By Lynne Frankenbery

How I Beat Crohn's

Through Diet Alone

By Lynne Frankenbery

Lynne Frankenbery

2019

First Printing: 2019

ISBN: 978-0-359-73427-6

Lynne Frankenbery

PO Box 104

Crescent, PA 15046-0104

www.HowIBeatCrohns-lynne.Blogspot.com

Special discounts are available on quantity purchases by corporations, associations, educators, and others. For details, contact the publisher at the above listed address.

U.S. trade bookstores and wholesalers: Please contact Lynne Frankenbery at lynne1408@earthlink.net.

This book is not intended to be a substitute for the medical advice of a licensed physician. The reader should consult a physician in any matters relating to his/her health.

*To my husband Ken and my daughters Aliah and Meghan.
Thank you for supporting me and encouraging me to finish this
book.*

Contents

Acknowledgements

I want to thank my daughter Aliah for helping me and encouraging me to write this book. Without you this book would not exist.

I also want to thank my family and friends including Ken, Meghan, Aunt Sandy, Uncle Harvey, Eric, Stephen, Shila, and Hilary. Thank you for supporting me through every stage of my disease and every struggle I faced. And thank you for your understanding and accommodating my needs by making changes in your cooking.

Thank you to all my doctors. Without you, I would not be here today. And thank you to those who donated their blood to me when I needed it the most.

Introduction

Approximately 700,000[1] people in the United States suffer from Crohn's disease, and in 2005 I became one of those people. Throughout my life, I had always tried to be healthy. Doing my best to take care of myself by eating right and exercising. Following my diagnosis, I was not looking forward to taking medication for the rest of my life. It was my belief that medicine was not the only approach to controlling this disease. So I searched for an alternative. After several years of working closely with my doctors, I found a different method that worked for me. And the best part was that no medications were needed. I found a way to beat my Crohn's disease through diet alone.

Some people would argue that diet has nothing to do with Crohn's disease. I might have believed that as well a few years ago. Until I discovered a clear connection between what I ate and how my body reacted. In the first half of this book, I talk about my own personal experiences learning to control my Crohn's and how I managed in my day-to-day life. The second half of the book is dedicated as a clear outline of how to identify foods that may be triggering Crohn's in an individual and how to tailor a diet based on personal dietary needs. Recipes are also included at the back of this book that are not only delicious but free from many common allergens.

Please be aware that I cannot claim to know the true cure for Crohn's disease but have personally found a diet that works best to control my disease. However, just because I found a specific diet that helped me beat my Crohn's does not mean my personal diet will work for someone else. Every person is different and the foods that trigger my Crohn's disease may be different than what triggers Crohn's in others.

Disclaimer:

I am not a doctor or a dietician. The information in this book is based on my own personal experiences and is in no way dietary advice on what someone else should or should not eat. Any desire to begin a new diet is a personal decision that is best made between a patient and a doctor. Please talk to your doctor before making any changes to your diet or changing/stopping medication.

What Is Crohn's Disease?

Crohn's disease is a chronic inflammatory condition of the digestive tract. The area most commonly affected is the end of the small bowel (ileum) and the colon. However, Crohn's can affect any region of the digestive system - from mouth to anus. While symptoms can vary, the most common include frequent diarrhea, bleeding, and abdominal pain and cramping. Widespread inflammation caused by Crohn's can even affect areas of the body not usually associated with the digestive tract, leading to inflammation of the skin, joints, and even eyes.[2]

Types of Crohn's

There are five types of Crohn's disease based on location and severity of the disease.

1. **Ileocolitis** - The most common type of Crohn's disease affects the colon and the ileum. The ileum is the region between the small intestines and the colon. Typical symptoms can include diarrhea, pain and/or cramping of the abdomen, and weight loss. It is estimated that nearly 45% of individuals diagnosed with Crohn's disease have Ileocolitis [3].
2. **Ileitis** - This type is similar to Ileocolitis; except only the ileum is affected. Symptoms are usually the same as with Ileocolitis -

diarrhea, abdominal pain and/or cramping, and weight loss. When Ileitis is severe, fistulas (inflammatory abscesses) can form in the abdomen. Ileitis makes up for 30% of Crohn's sufferers [3].

3. **Jejunoileitis** - The middle part of the small intestines is affected by this type of Crohn's disease. Symptoms include cramps following meals, diarrhea, fistulas, and intense abdomen pain. This form is fairly uncommon in individuals diagnosed with Crohn's.

4. **Gastroduodenal Crohn's** - This type causes damage to the stomach and duodenum (first part of the small intestines). Common symptoms include nausea, vomiting, and loss of appetite.

5. **Crohn's (Granulomatous) colitis** - This type of Crohn's affects mostly the colon. Common symptoms include bleeding, diarrhea, joint pain, ulcers, and fistulas [4]. I was diagnosed with this type of Crohn's.

Symptoms of Crohn's

While the symptoms mentioned above for the different types of Crohn's are the common symptoms most people will get, Crohn's can cause many other symptoms. These include abdomen pain, diarrhea, bleeding, fatigue, weight loss, fever, night sweats, lack of appetite, joint pain, anemia, skin rashes, and more. Symptoms can range from mild to severe. Some symptoms, such as bleeding and dehydration, can even become so severe that hospitalization is needed [5]. To summarize, you end up feeling like crap and spending way too much time on a porcelain throne. Having Crohn's can be life inhibiting. It affects your social life. How can you go out and enjoy yourself when you need to plan your day around the bathroom?

How Crohn's is Diagnosed

There is no definitive test for Crohn's. Diagnosis is based on several different tests and symptoms so a doctor will usually order a combination of tests to get a complete picture of the situation. An x-ray is sometimes taken to look for narrowing in the colon. If the colon becomes too narrow it can lead to obstructions. A CT scan is used to look for abscesses, bleeding ulcers, and fistulas. Any blockages in the colon can also be shown using a CT scan. An MRI will sometimes be used to show the inflamed tissues in more detail [6].

Doctors will often want to perform an endoscopy and colonoscopy before making a diagnosis. This involves using a small camera attached to a flexible tube to view the insides of the stomach and colon. With an endoscopy, the tube is inserted through the mouth and down into the stomach. Thankfully, the patient is asleep for this. For a colonoscopy, the tube is inserted through the anus and up into the colon. The patient is usually in a twilight state of consciousness during this process. More recently, there are now video capsule endoscopies and colonoscopies. In these cases, a tiny camera is placed in a capsule which can then be swallowed. The camera takes pictures as it travels through the digestive tract [7].

Blood tests are also often very helpful to prove if there is any inflammation in the body, infection, or anemia.

Causes of Crohn's

There is no known cause of Crohn's disease, although several factors seem to be involved. Most experts believe Crohn's is caused by a combination of changes to the immune system, presence of specific bacteria in the body, genetic factors, and environmental triggers.

5

The immune system is believed to trigger the inflammation associated with Crohn's. Inflammation is actually the body's way of limiting the spread of a foreign substance, bacteria, or virus. Although the true trigger for the disease is not known for certain, scientists believe it may be due to an overreaction of the immune system, possibly attacking something that is not really there [9]. However, it is my belief that there may be something there that we don't see but the body does.

There is also a genetic connection. People who are of Jewish Ashkenazi descent, which I am, seem more prone to Crohn's. It seems to affect both genders equally. Diagnosis is most common between the ages of 15 and 35 but can happen at any age [8]. I was already 43 when I was diagnosed.

There may be some connection to the environment. Crohn's tends to be more common in industrialized countries. This may be because of the high consumption of processed foods [10]. Our food supply is getting further and further away from the farm. Even when we try to eat healthy foods such as fruits and vegetables, unless they are grown organically, we have to worry about pesticide use. What is healthy anyhow?

There is now also evidence that smoking may make Crohn's disease worse. There have been studies done that show a connection [11].

Complications of Crohn's

Depending on the severity and length of illness, Crohn's can cause a whole host of complications. For example, ulcers that form in the digestive tract can bleed and even lead to infection, becoming severe enough to make surgery necessary.

The more inflammation that the colon undergoes, the higher the risk for colon and small intestine cancer [13]. This is why it is so necessary to reduce the inflammation.

Obstructions can lead to a condition called megacolon. Nothing can move through the colon so everything gets backed up. There is no movement and the colon become swollen. The colon literally becomes giant or mega. This can be a life threatening situation.

Because of the inflammation, Crohn's patients may not be able to absorb nutrients such as B12 and vitamin D. This can lead to weight and bone loss. Likewise, severe bleeding can lead to anemia, sometimes necessitating a blood transfusion [14]. I once had bleeding that was so severe I had to have a blood transfusion in February 2008. We are talking about a lot of blood loss.

Treatments

Though there is no cure, there are several classes of drugs that are used to treat the symptoms of Crohn's disease. These include antibiotics, aminosalicylates, corticosteroids, immune modifiers, and biological therapies.

For milder cases, some relief may be found with over the counter medications, such as antidiarrheals, pain relievers and vitamins [15].

Antibiotics such as Metronidazole and Ciprofloxacin are generally prescribed. Though they are usually well tolerated, they may cause side effects such as nausea and diarrhea. They cannot be taken long term and may mess up the delicate balance of good bacteria in the gut.

Aminosalicylates can be administered orally or rectally. These drugs are used to calm and soothe the colon. The oral form is designed to bypass the stomach and therefore distribute medicine on the intestinal wall.

Immune modifiers work by suppressing the immune system. It is the immune system that triggers the inflammation to protect the body from invasion. The inflammation will then be reduced. However, with the immune system suppressed it weakens the body's ability to fight infections. This may cause problems with other infections popping up.

A new and promising treatment is fecal transplantation. Healthy fecal material is transferred from one person to another. Gross as it may sound it has proven to be somewhat successful.

Constant inflammation and bleeding can lead to ulcers, fistulas, obstructions, and more. These can become so severe that medicine is not enough, making surgery necessary. Sixty to seventy-five percent of Crohn's patients will need to have surgery at some point in their life [16].

There are several types of surgery depending on the location and the severity of the inflammation [17]. Stricture-plasty is a surgery used to widen an opening in the colon. No tissue is removed during this process. A resection removes portions of the intestinal. In the most of severe cases, a proctocolectomy or colectomy removes the rectum as well as a whole or part of the colon.

The Early Years

My entire life seems to have been moving in one direction. I have always seen food as a way to nurture the body as well as a way to bring family together. I have literally spent many years studying nutrition and learning healthy ways to cook. From early on, I realized that what I ate had a huge impact on my health and how I felt.

One of my earliest memories of food was when I was about six years old. I remember wanting to eat canned spinach every day for lunch. Seems like an odd craving. Around the same time I was drinking a lot of milk and not much else. I came down with milk anemia. I wondered now if my spinach craving was due to my iron deficiency. I even remember my father mentioning this as a possibility. Even at that young age I could understand what my dad was saying about craving something that my body needed. Just like craving water when we are thirsty. I was possibly craving the iron from the spinach.

My family was a little different for the time in the 1960s. We were always into "health food" and didn't believe that popping a prescription pill was the cure-all. The 1970s were the start of the holistic and natural medicine craze but my family was a little ahead of the times.

That's not to say that we were against standard health care. We understood the need of going to the doctor when we got sick. We took our antibiotics and got our vaccines. We followed the doctor's orders. I'd still go to the doctor and take medicines and such when we needed to, but my family was still big on natural cures and supplements for a lot of problems.

My mom used to have a subscription to *Prevention* magazine. They would always be talking about the newest holistic products and healthy diets. We were always trying out healthy and tasty recipes and my mother loved trying out new products. She would always be ordering different supplements and vitamins; even letting my brother and I pick out some products we wanted.

When we were teens, my brother ended up working at a local health food store. He would sometimes bring home the weirdest new supplements for us to try. I remember trying out chewable protein tablets, wheat germ oil, dolomite, and even desiccated liver! It might sound crazy to think about now, but there were the hot new items at the time. Granola was making a huge impact in the 70s and I got to try it for the first time as a teen.

It was my brother who first introduced us to fresh juicing when he brought home a juicer one day. Unlike today, organic fruits and vegetables were not as readily available and were terribly expensive when they were. So we used mostly non-organic/commercial veggies. We limited pesticides by peeling skins and washing everything thoroughly. My family loved to try all sorts of new and delicious juice combos. I loved that these juices tasted so good and gave me a great boost of energy!

As I got older, I would try different cleanses, such as just eating vegetables, along with various herbal supplements, juices or just apples. A cleanse is supposed to work by giving your digestive tract a break. Nothing but juice and water or certain fruits and vegetables is consumed for a few days giving your body a little vacation. During this break your body is able to do some internal cleaning that it otherwise may not have had a chance to do while it was digesting food. I tried it several times. It's also hard to believe, but as a child the only place I could find yogurt was at a health food store. Yogurt wouldn't be found in any modern grocery store until the late 1970s. I used to frequent health food stores to buy yogurts for myself all the time. It was a huge craze at the time for being plentiful in good bacteria, something very important for a healthy colon.

Like a lot of younger people these days, I went through a vegetarian phase as a teen. Being a vegetarian was already a rare fringe trend for the time, and almost no one had even heard of the term 'vegan'. I decided to become a vegetarian for the health benefits that people were talking about and it seemed like a good and healthy idea. Well, my journey into vegetarianism lasted for only six months. There wasn't a lot of information around about being a vegetarian and there weren't many good choices out there for a healthy diet, especially in restaurants. And although my family was fairly supportive of my decision, they still ate meat. I remember sitting at the breakfast table some mornings and watching as they munched on crunchy and delicious bacon, all the while my mouth watering. So long story short, my vegetarian diet didn't last very long and I ended up giving it up.

Just like my brother, I ended up working at a local health food store in my 20s. My manager was great and had a passion for health foods and supplements, and she would always by encouraging me to learn more about the products and how they could help people. In between customers I would read the books and magazines they carried which carried a wealth of information. In this time I learned a huge amount about nutrition, herbal medicine, and holistic healing.

In addition to diet, I exercised my whole life. I ran, played tennis and basketball as a teenager. I walked to and from the university campus every day. And I stopped at the track on the way home to run a few miles. I got really into yoga in my 20s. I was thin, fit and active.

In short, I tried my best to eat healthy and live a healthy life. But then things changed when I was 43. I was diagnosed with Crohn's disease. I thought that only people who lived unhealthy lifestyles came down with diseases. After living such a healthy lifestyle, how could this even be possible? Because of the way I was raised, always looking for a natural alternative to medicine, I was motivated to search for another way.

Discovering I Had Crohn's

Looking back to right before I was diagnosed with Crohn's, I remember that it didn't happen all of a sudden although it seemed that way at the time.

Before my diagnosis, I didn't really have any health problems. I liked to think that I was fairly healthy and my colon seemed fine. No problems whatsoever.

I woke up one morning thinking that it would be a normal day like any other. But after I went to the bathroom and saw blood, I hate to say, but I didn't actually give it much thought. I'd just keep an eye on it. Probably just a one time thing. It was probably nothing.

The next day there was blood again, but this time a bit more. Well, it's still not much to worry about. I'll probably be better by tomorrow.

The third morning came around and... nothing. No blood, no stool. Nothing at all, which honestly wasn't *great* but not *bad* either. Just a little constipated but it will pass.

The fourth day came, and nothing.

The fifth day came, and nothing.

The sixth day, seventh, eighth, and ninth day... and nothing.

Not one bowel movement for more than a whole week. I was more constipated than I could ever remember being. My stomach was hurting and starting to bloat.

And don't think that I didn't try to fix things during that week. I did, I tried everything. I tried prunes, olive oil, even laxatives weren't working. Nothing was working so I made an appointment with my doctor. This wasn't normal constipation.

This first thing my doctor did was send me for a colonoscopy. But I was only 43 and had never had one before. Most people don't get one done until they're around 50. Suffice it to say, I was feeling more than apprehensive. Fear struck me as I started to wonder about what the doctor would find. Was this the beginning of something really bad? Did I have colon cancer? Would I need surgery? What was going to happen? I was so scared and had no clue what to expect. My imagination was running wild with everything it could possibly be.

The day before the colonoscopy I took the prep. Back then they were still using the phospho-soda bottles that are bad for the kidneys. It was really salty. It was pretty harsh too. Today's preps are much more gentle. Well, the prep got me going and very clean. Mind you I had been backed up for over a week. It was quite a relief.

The day of my colonoscopy I remember sitting in my doctor's office with shaky hands and a knot in my throat. I had no idea what to expect when this was over and my imagination wasn't helping.

The nurses got me prepped with an IV and gave me a drug to calm me and put me in a twilight state for the procedure. I would be relaxed and out of it, but not fully asleep.

I have a vague memory of "waking up" during the colonoscopy to my doctor saying, "There it is!" Facing the screen used to look inside the colon I remember seeing a lot of blood! Yikes! Of course, I didn't know the ramification of this and just thought the worst.

The rest of the procedure was a blur. However, I do remember talking to the doctor afterwards. He said that he found ulcers in my colon which explained the bleeding. He also told me that my terminal ileum had swollen shut. That was why I was not able to have bowel movements. The terminal ileum is like a doorway between the small intestines and the colon. My diagnosis was Crohn's disease.

They put me on steroids to calm the inflammation and Pentasa (an anti-inflammatory) to help prevent future flares. They also had me take mineral oil to prevent the constipation. These medications would treat my symptoms, but there was no curing my Crohn's. I was still bleeding a bit, but feeling fairly okay physically.

But emotionally I felt victimized. I didn't do anything wrong and then this just came out of the blue. I felt like I didn't have any control over the situation. My cousin had been diagnosed with Crohn's but she was the only one I knew of.

I felt isolated and overwhelmed. I was a single mother with two young daughters. Would Crohn's affect my ability to take care of them? As a single mother I already felt like I sometimes didn't have enough time or energy some days. I certainly didn't have time to be going to the bathroom 20 times a day, while taking care of small children.

I didn't have much of support system in the beginning. Back then, there weren't many forums or blogs online with people like me talking about how they were handling similar problems and who understood what I was going through.

I realize that not everyone reacts that same way after getting a diagnoses like this. Some people are shocked, angry, filled with denial early on. What I did feel was defeated and depressed. It felt like a slap in the face after all I had done to try and stay healthy. All the years of eating healthy and exercising did nothing.

This was the first time I had to take a daily medicine and it made me feel like I was failing. I was getting older and my body wasn't working like it should anymore. It was frustrating and I was feeling anxious about my future. I had recently started a new relationship and was worried about how my diagnosis could interfere with our intimacy.

The Bad Years

After my diagnosis I did what most people might do and that was to listen to the doctor. They started me on a fairly high dose of steroids (Prednisone) and an anti-inflammatory (Pentasa). At first I was feeling great! The bleeding stopped completely and because of the steroids I felt full of energy. I was having normal bowel movements and the inflammation was gone. No bleeding, bloating, cramping, diarrhea or exhaustion.

I was feeling great. I had lots of energy and felt like I could do anything. I wasn't going to the bathroom all the time (before I was going about 20 times per day). It was a welcome relief. Unfortunately steroids are only a short term medicine and can't be taken for a long time. I was worried of the consequences of going off of them because steroids were what had helped me stop bleeding in the first place. I was worried that when I stopped the steroids the bleeding would come back. But for now I was taking them on a regular basis. It was a relief to have a social life again and be able to go out and have the freedom that I used to have. I was feeling hopeful again that I would be able to take control of my disease.

After several weeks of being on steroids, I was starting to get bloated. My tummy and even my face looked swollen. I gained weight around my chin and jaw area. This was what's known as 'moon-face' [18]. I also started gaining weight overall. Well, not too bad of a tradeoff considering I wasn't bleeding anymore. But the bloating and weight gain didn't get better. It was getting worse and I was disappointed that the steroids, the same pill that helped me so much physically, would hurt me just as much emotionally. I felt fat and I felt ugly. The bloating and weight gain were symptoms that were having a big impact on my appearance that I had no control over. I was worried that I would have to be on and off of steroids for the rest of my life. I didn't want to settle for dealing with these symptoms. They were seriously affecting my social life. I had just started a new relationship with Ken, who is now my husband. It affected my confidence. I remember going to a banquet with him but I almost canceled because of the bloating around my face. I felt embarrassed and self-conscious. I was apprehensive to see him that day but when I did, he made me feel like I looked okay. He was very sweet. About a year later I married him.

After a few months, my doctors wanted me to wean off of the steroids. Apparently it is not good to stay on steroids too long. It can deplete calcium out of your bones, put strain on your adrenal glands (adrenaline), and lower your immunity [4]. Easier said than done. As I lowered the dosage, I began to lose energy. However, I was also shedding the weight. I was happy that I was losing the weight from the steroids. But once I got down to about 15 milligrams I started bleeding again. My doctors had me bouncing up and down in milligrams, as I would start or stop bleeding. Finally I made myself get off because this is what the doctors wanted, but I would still bleed. I also had lots of inflammation both in my colon and even in my joints what made them feel achy and sometimes painful.

One of the hardest things about Crohn's disease for me was dealing with fatigue. Feeling tired after a long and busy day is a normal type of fatigue. But the fatigue that comes with Crohn's disease is different. No amount of sleep will make you feel better. It's constant and debilitating. Since I was off steroids and was bleeding again, I eventually ended up getting anemia. This caused me to feel even more fatigue throughout the day. My legs felt so weak, like I was walking through water or like they were made of jelly. My head felt like it was stuffed full of cotton and everything was foggy.

I was feeling depressed and lost. I tried searching for solution that didn't include steroids but I was feeling hopeless. The medicine I was on wasn't working and I was afraid that I would stay sick. Most days were not good, either bleeding, diarrhea, constipation, or just overall exhaustion.

Making the Connection

Early 2006 I started to notice a pattern. Some days seemed to be pretty good and other days seemed a lot worse. By 'pretty good' I don't mean that these days were at all perfect, I mean that I had fairly normal bowel movements and minimal bleeding. So as far as good and bad days went, I started to ask myself what made the difference? Was it stress? Was it something I ate? My doctors said that the differences weren't related to food.

Despite what my doctors said, I wanted to be sure for myself that food wasn't causing me problems so I started a food diary. Pretty soon I began to notice that there was a pattern when I ate gluten and the severity of my symptoms. I remember the day that I finally figured out the connection for myself. It had been a pretty bad day for me and I was feeling very sick with lots of blood and diarrhea. But I remember that the day before I had made some whole-wheat carrot muffins. Thinking that there might be a link there, I did some more research. Looking back in my journal, I noticed that I would always get gas that day after eating wheat or gluten. When I ate a lot of gluten, like spaghetti or bread, a few hours later there would be lots of gas. I always liked to call myself the pasta queen because I loved pasta sooo much and I ate it all the time. Some days were worse than others depending on how much wheat/gluten I had eaten.

So I worked on eliminating all wheat, gluten and wheat/gluten derivatives from my diet. I wanted to see for sure if this was what was causing my to flare, and I found pretty good results! Completely cutting out gluten caused my Crohn's to drastically improve. I wasn't flaring as badly or as often. But it only helped about 85%. I still had some symptoms but they were a lot milder than they used to be. However I wasn't getting symptoms every day. My flares began to get more spread out and milder. When I did experience a flare, it was not nearly as severe.

I knew that I was on to something and with my new diet I had begun to feel a lot better. A few weeks after going off gluten, I went for a follow-up visit with my doctor. She wanted to see how I was doing with my medications. I had asked her about going off gluten and while she said that Crohn's disease was not food related, I was welcome to try by changing my diet.

A few months go by and my diet was still working. It still wasn't perfect and I was still flaring, but it was a lot less severe. When Christmas came around I remember getting a great treat as a gift from a friend of mine. It was one of those flavored popcorn tins with buttered, caramel, and kettle corn. They were so good and I'll admit I probably ate more than I should have in one day! But it was the holidays and I was celebrating. Well, the day after Christmas was bad for me. Really…bad. I flared so badly that I ended up calling my doctor and got put back on steroids. According to one of my nurses, these sort of problems happened a lot around the Holidays for other people too.

A few weeks later, my colon was back under control with the help of the steroids. One day I was invited to dinner with my fiancé's family. I was going to meet some of his relatives for the first time so I was a bit nervous. We had a delicious meal, prepared by my future mother in-law. It was ham, potatoes and corn. I don't eat corn very often, but it was yummy. That night my stomach made so much noise!

And then in the morning I had another bad flare.

At this point I thought that maybe corn was causing me to flare. Could corn really be causing me more problems? Gluten is one thing but corn is as American as apple pie. Corn is a tradition, just a vegetable. This didn't seem to be right but I figured I would try and find out. Three days after cutting out all corn products, my flares stopped. Completely. No gluten and no corn. My colon's health was at 100%. I couldn't believe it!

It took me a long time to make the connections but it was worth it. I now know which foods are safe for me to eat. I had several months worth of food diaries. I went over them again and again to find the solution and as I refined my diet, I felt better and better. Later on I give a sample of what a typical diary might look like and provide tips on how to make food connections. This is a long process, but so worthwhile.

The Big Flare

For the next few years after discovering that gluten and corn were causing my Crohn's flares, I had been doing really well. For the most part my colon was fine and I was healthy. The only time I ever bled or had diarrhea anymore was when I made a mistake with my diet by eating something containing gluten, corn, or one of their derivatives. Even when I did flare it was much more minor and easy to control. My doctors took me off all medicines and I was doing good.

Unfortunately, my health took a turn for the worse in February 2008. I had caught the flu that year and it was the first time I was that sick since being diagnosed. I was running a bad fever and had been getting a little diarrhea, but it wasn't so bad because at first there was no bleeding. But after several days of running a fever on and off, I began to flare. It was the biggest flare that I could ever remember having and I was bleeding severely.

It was the flare that couldn't be controlled. I hadn't eaten any gluten or corn that would have upset my colon, but the stress of the flu must have been a trigger which I had no way to stop. My fiancee had caught the flu that same year but it didn't hit him as badly. He was still able to help take care of me and watch my daughters. He was a life-saver. But, over the course of those days I had lost way too much blood. I ended up being hospitalized for four days before I was considered healthy enough to go home. The doctors put me on a strong dose of steroids that helped to immediately put me back into remission and stop the bleeding. But I was still anemic after bleeding so badly and had to get a blood transfusion to get my red blood cell count up again.

My hospitalization happened in February and I was planning on getting married in April. The steroids I was on caused me to bloat again and I had major ulcers that were still causing me problems after my release from the hospital. I was worried that I would still be having problems for my wedding. Would I still enjoy the honeymoon or would I be stuck in a bathroom for most of it?

With all the bloating and getting 'moon-face' again, I was worried about how I might look for the wedding. I tried not to feel too insecure about it but that's easier said than done. I didn't feel very attractive and was always upset about how my 'moon-face' looked. But my fiancee Ken was wonderful

In March, one month before the wedding, I remember going to the photographer to plan for the wedding and I couldn't help but worry how the photos would turn out. A few weeks before the wedding, after I had gained weight and was bloated from the steroids, I had to go to a seamstress to adjust the dress, since I had gained weight. She did what she could but there wasn't a lot of material to work with. The dress ended up still being too tight. On my wedding day I had to squeeze in with the help of my bridesmaid and it was so tight that I could barely breathe. I had "back cleavage". I felt like those women that wore corsets and I was scared that I would pass out because my dress was so tight.

As it turned out, I was worrying for nothing and the wedding was wonderful!

Food Diary

The way that I found out what foods were causing my flares was through keeping a food diary. I wrote down everything that I ate or drank. Literally everything. Even mints, gum, and seasonings were noted. I noted the brands of all the foods since different brands have different ingredients.

Then on the same page I would write down how I felt that day. Was I feeling tired or energetic? I noted the highlights of my day and whether or not I was feeling stressed.

Now there is no tactful way to say this, I also recorded every time I went to the bathroom and a general description of each bowel movement. TMI? Maybe, and I know this may sound a little gross but it was a vital part of the process that helped me figure out what was triggering my flares.

If I had a particularly bad day I was able to look back in my diary to see what I had eaten the previous day. Sometimes I could see certain trends. Sometimes I couldn't figure anything out at all. It was when I did start to see a pattern, specifically when I ate gluten and corn, that it started to make a difference.

Keeping a diary was also helpful when I had a particularly good day. I would look back on what I had eaten the previous day to note "safe" foods. If I had eaten a food and the results were good, I would repeat the food after a while to see if the results were still good.

This was a long process but well worth the effort. Once I was able to start making connections I was slowly able to clean up my diet of trigger foods, or foods that made me flare. The longer I kept track, the better my results. Below I have a sample of a food diary. Everyone is different. This is meant only as a guide.

March 5, 2019

Breakfast:
- 2 hard boiled eggs
- 1 slice of toast (circle K brand)
-   with butter (Bluebonnet)
- Tea (with sugar)

Lunch:
- Pepsi (regular)
- 3 slices pizza (with pepperoni and mushrooms) (pizza shop)

Dinner:
- Homemade lemonade (with sugar)
- Grilled salmon (with salt, pepper, and lemon)
- French fries (Oreda)
- Ketchup (Heinz)
- Steamed broccoli

Dessert:
- 2 chocolate chip cookies (bakery)
- Milk (2%)

Snacks:
- Strawberries
- Three Musketeers candy bar

Bowel Movements:
- 7:00 am. BM (high blood)
- 8:00 am. Blood only, no stool
- 10:00 am. Bloody diarrhea, medium blood
- 11:30 am. BM, medium blood
- 3:00 am. Blood only

Notes:
- Cramps all day
- Low energy
- Took a nap (2 hours)
- Worked 9 to 12

March 6, 2019

Breakfast:
- Tea (with sugar)
- White rice with lentils
- Orange

Lunch:
Cucumber Sandwich
- 2 slices gluten free bread (Against the Grain)

- Cucumber
- Mozzarella cheese
- Vegan mayo
- Broccoli sprouts

Dinner:
- Roasted chicken (with salt and pepper)
- Apple juice
- Roasted potatoes

Dessert:
- 2 Hershey Kisses

Snacks:
- Cocoa loco bar (gluten free)

Other:
- 2 Liquid Advil (headache)

Bowel Movements:
- 3:00 am. Bloody diarrhea
- 5:00 am. Bloody diarrhea
- 6:30 am. Bloody diarrhea
- 7:30 am. Small stool, lots of gas, high blood
- 9:00 am. Small stool, very high blood
- 11:00 am. Small stool, medium blood
- Afternoon. No stools

Notes:
- Felt ill all morning, afternoon was better
- Thirsty all day
- Couldn't do homework with kids
- Took a nap (2 hours)
- A little nauseous

There are many things that can be learned just by looking at these few examples. In terms of food affecting the colon, food passes through fairly quickly. It only takes at most two days to note the results of a particular food. When foods do flare up the colon, it also doesn't take long for the flare to resolve itself. Keeping a food diary helped me to be able to look back on the previous day to learn about what I had eaten

On the first day of this imaginary diary, I ate toast and pizza. Lots of gluten. I noted that the next day was very bad with lots of bleeding. It could have been from the wheat flour in the pizza. Or it could have been from something else. Was it the cheese on the pizza? Maybe it was the pizza sauce? There were so many possible causes.

So the next day, I tried gluten free. I had rice and potatoes, but no breads, except the gluten free one. I also avoided any sauces on my chicken. I still felt ill during the morning because the day before there had been a lot of gluten. The afternoon I started to feel better. I will tell you that the following day was very good. It can work that quickly.

I noticed that on the second day I was wheat and corn free. It was followed by a good day. I noted that the Against the Grain breads do not flare me. I also noted that cheese was not the culprit either. I took Advil (liquid) for my head, but it did not affect my colon. Even medicines were recorded.

Through this process, my diet got tweaked every day. This was a long process. I would try foods and note the results. I would try to repeat good days with similar foods. After a while I had it down almost to a science.

Of course I also made mistakes along the way. Sometimes I was too hungry and ate things without checking the label. Sometimes I didn't realize that a particular ingredient was derived from corn or wheat. Eating in restaurants was also taking a big chance. I could never be sure of all the ingredients.

Corn and wheat were my triggers. This was clear. I also found out that corn and wheat derivatives were also triggers. These are ingredients that come from corn or wheat, but with the names they sometimes go by you would never know it. Food derivatives are discussed in the next chapter.

In a later chapter I talk about the 'Elimination Diet' and how it is helpful when trying to recognize trigger foods. Remember, everyone is different. My triggers were corn and wheat. Other people may have dairy or soy as a trigger. Other common allergens are fish, peanuts, tree nuts, and eggs. The important thing was that I had to figure out what they were so I could get back to feeling healthy.

Food Intolerances vs. Food Allergies

It is at this point that I would like to have a brief discussion on food intolerances versus food allergies. While they share some similarities, food allergies are often more severe and can sometimes be life threatening. Food intolerances are generally milder than food allergies and are not normally life threatening, although they can be, and can require hospital treatment. While a food intolerance mostly affects the digestive tract, food allergies affect the entire body, including the immune system [19].

Food allergies come on suddenly, usually soon after a food is eaten. The body reacts immediately. Unlike with allergies, food intolerances may take several hours or even days to affect the body. As for the colon, it may take several hours until the offending food reaches the intestines and thereby irritate it. By the time symptoms show up, several different meals and foods may have been eaten. It may take as long as 48 hours to show up [20].

When someone has a food allergy they will get a reaction every time they eat the food. And it doesn't matter how small of an amount they eat, they will get a reaction. This is what makes it so dangerous for them to eat out. Contrarily, food intolerances may not happen every time. It may depend on how much of the offending food is eaten [21].

The symptoms of food intolerances affect mostly the digestive tract, such as diarrhea, bloating, nausea, abdominal pain, vomiting and heartburn. Though there are some other symptoms of food intolerances that can affect other area as well, such as headaches and fatigue. The symptoms of food allergies are more severe as they can affect the entire body including the digestive, immune, and cardiovascular system [22]. This is why food allergies area so life threatening They can make it difficult for the person to breath and they can go into cardiac arrest.

Food Derivatives

Food derivatives are things that are derived from other foods. There are many derivatives that are made from gluten. One example of this is malt. Malt is a derivative of barley. Barley is glutinous and therefore malt is also considered glutinous. The list of food derivatives for gluten are exhaustive.

I noticed very early on that I had to eliminate not only gluten and corn from my diet, but also all of their derivatives. Eliminating all the derivatives from my diet was absolutely the key for me. Ingredients such as cornstarch, corn syrup and maltodextrin all had to be eliminated in order to achieve remission. I have heard of people not having good results when eliminating gluten from their diet. But it does make me wonder if they were still getting gluten from these derivatives.

Below is a list of foods that contain gluten or its derivatives. This list is by no means complete, but will give a good idea of where gluten is usually found [23].

- Barley
- Bagels
- Baking soda
- Beer
- Brewer's yeast
- Brown rice syrup
- Bulgur (whole wheat)

- Buns
- Cake
- Caramel coloring
- Cereal
- Cookies
- Couscous
- Crackers

- Dextrin
- Donuts
- Durum wheat (found in pasta)
- Farino
- Faro
- Fermented grain extract
- Flying fish eggs
- Food coloring
- Graham flour
- Hydrolyzed malt extract
- Hydrolyzed vegetable protein
- Kanut
- Licorice
- Malt
- Malted milk
- Malt extract
- Malt syrup
- Malt flavoring
- Malt vinegar (potato chips)
- Matzo
- Modified starch
- Muffins
- Natural flavor
- Oatmeal
- Pancakes
- Pie crust
- Rice, flavored
- Rye
- Rye beer
- Rye bread
- Soy sauce
- Seitan
- Semolina (pasta)
- Soup
- Spelt
- Tacos
- Tortillas
- Triticale
- Waffles
- Wheat
- Wheat berries
- Wheat bran
- Wheat germ
- Wheat starch
- Whole wheat
- Yeast extract

Listed below are some other possible sources of gluten [24]. These ingredients may or may not contain gluten so I try to avoid these unless I am very sure of the sources.

- Anti-caking agents
- Baked beans (canned)
- Chutneys
- Dextrin

- Edible starch
- Emulsifiers
- Fillers
- Gum base
- Homeopathic remedies
- Hydrolyzed proteins
- Instant coffee
- Lunch meats
- Modified food starch
- Mono and diglycerides
- Mustard
- Natural flavoring
- Non dairy creamer
- Spices (especially curry)
- Stamps and envelopes (when you lick them)
- Tabouleh
- Textured vegetable protein
- Turkey (pre-basted)
- Vegetable gum
- White and malt vinegar
- Vitamin E oil
- White pepper

In addition, here are some derivatives and hidden sources of corn: [25] [26]

- Aspartame
- Ascorbic acid (vitamin C)
- Beans, canned
- Calcium citrate
- Caramel
- Cellulose
- Citric Acid
- Corn flakes
- Corn meal
- Corn starch
- Golden syrup
- High fructose corn syrup
- Hominy
- Iodized salt
- Ketchup
- Lecithin
- Maize
- Malt
- Maltodextrin
- Malitol
- Mayonnaise
- Microcrystalline cellulose
- Modified corn starch
- Modified food starch
- MSG
- Mustard
- Pickles
- Popcorn
- Powdered sugar
- Relish

- Sorbitol
- Splenda
- Vanilla
- White distilled vinegar
- Xanthan gum
- Zein

Another common allergen that may cause flares in some people is dairy. I do not actually flare from dairy. I do limit it however because I am lactose intolerant. Luckily there are plenty of substitutes and I like to drink Lactaid milk and use it in all my recipes. The following list shows sources of milk and dairy products [27]. Once again, this list is not exhaustive as dairy is found everywhere.

- Buttermilk
- Bean curd
- Baby soy formula
- Caseinate
- Cottage cheese
- Cream
- Cream cheese
- Ghee
- Half and half
- Ice cream
- Lactose
- Milk (of any kind including whole, skim, 2%, condensed, evaporated, goat, malted, chocolate, strawberry, acidophilus)
- Milk protein
- Milk sugar
- Cheese (all including Edam, Brie, Gouda, Havarti, muenster, mozzarella, etc.)
- Chocolate
- Cottage cheese
- Curds
- Custard
- Margarine
- Mayonnaise
- Pudding
- Sour cream
- Whey
- Whipped cream
- Yogurt

Another common allergen many people are sensitive with is soy. Here are some places that soy is usually found. Again, this is not a complete list, but does give an idea of how prevalent soy is in our foods [28].

- Edamame
- Kinako flour (made from roasted soy beans)
- Soya
- Soy albumin
- Soy beans
- Soy cheese
- Soy fiber
- Soy flour
- Soy granules
- Soy grits
- Soy lecithin
- Soy milk
- Soy nuts
- Soy oil
- Soy protein
- Soy sprouts
- Soy yogurt
- Tamari
- Tempeh
- Teriyaki sauce
- Textured vegetable protein
- Tofu

Other Common allergens include eggs, fish, shellfish, peanuts, tree nuts.

The Elimination Diet

One way to determine which foods may be a problem is to use the Elimination Diet. There are basically two ways to approach the elimination diet. The first way is to eliminate everything in your diet except really safe foods and then slowly add foods back. The other approach is to eliminate one type of food at a time [29]. The first approach is quick but very hard to stick to. The second approach takes weeks or months to have an effect but is easier to stick with. I decided to use the second approach.

The first approach to the elimination diet is to eliminate all possible foods that could be a problem. These may be wheat, gluten, corn, milk, fish, citric acid, nuts, soy, and eggs. It doesn't leave a whole lot of foods that are considered safe. A person may be able to eat plain rice and vegetables with some meat. Maybe gluten free spaghetti with sauce. The choices would be quite limited and this could work for some people that don't mind a stricter diet.

With the second approach to the elimination diet, one food type is eliminated at a time to see what the effects are. This is where the food diary comes in and why it is so important. I started by eliminating wheat and gluten. This is probably a good place to start. I was able to tell within days if a particular food had been causing problems. For me, giving up wheat and gluten helped about 85%. I still avoided wheat and gluten but then, in addition, I eliminated corn and corn derivatives. It was then that I was able to achieve 100% remission.

The Specific Carbohydrate Diet (SCD)

The Specific Carbohydrate Diet (SCD) was formulated by Sidney Haas, M.D. as a way to treat her 5 year old daughter who had Ulcerative Colitis [34]. There has been some evidence that this diet can actually help to put Ulcerative Colitis and even Crohn's disease sufferers in remission. There was a study done at Seattle Children's Hospital which looked at the effect of diet alone on children with Crohn's disease. Most of them were able to achieve remission [35].

During the time that I was formulating my diet, I had never even heard of the SCD. I was simply noting which foods would flare me and which foods were safe. Interestingly enough, these two diets are very similar.

Despite being similar, both diets were created in two very different ways. The SCD eliminates complex carbohydrates in order to give the gut a break and therefore help heal itself. In contrast, my diet eliminates gluten, corn, and all derivatives of gluten and corn, since they appear to trigger inflammation in my colon.

While the SCD eliminates complex carbs like wheat and corn, it is much more restrictive than my diet. For example, I still eat starches and beans such as potatoes and chickpeas. These starchy foods are not allowed on the SCD.

Either way, there is enough agreement between these two diets to warrant a review. Two different approaches that can lead to the same results. Below is a general chart comparing foods that are allowed on the SCD and foods that I allow. This chart does not, of course, contain every single food, but it does give a general idea.

Grains and Seeds:

Food	SCD	My Diet
Wheat	No	No
Rice	No	Yes
Oats	No	Yes - Gluten Free oats
Millet	No	Yes
Barley	No	No
Rye	No	No
Quinoa	No	Yes
Tapioca	No	Yes
Buckwheat	No	Yes
Amaranth	No	Yes
Flaxseed	No	Yes
Chia Seeds	No	Yes
Sunflower Seeds	Yes	Yes
Sesame Seeds	Yes	Yes
Pumpkin Seeds	Yes	Yes

Fruits and Vegetables:

Food	SCD	My Diet
Canned Fruits	Yes - If made with natural fruit juices only	Yes - If made with real sugar or natural fruit juices
Canned Vegetables	No	Yes
Starchy Vegetables (ex: potatoes, carrots, peas and yams, taro)	No	Yes
Pickled Vegetables (with sugar)	No	No
Corn	No	No
Seaweed Products	No	Yes

Dairy:

Food	SCD	My Diet
Milk	No	Yes
Non-Dairy Milks (ex: Almond, Rice, Soy)	No	Yes
Natural Cheese	No	Yes - If free of corn starch

Dairy (cont.):

Food	SCD	My Diet
Processed Cheese	No	Yes - If free of corn starch
Cottage Cheese	No	Yes - If free of vinegar
Sour Cream	No	Yes - If free of vinegar
Cream Cheese	No	Yes - If free of xanthan gum
Butter	No	Yes
Margarine	No	Yes - If free of corn oil
Yogurt	No	Yes - If free of cornstarch and corn syrup
Ice Cream	No	Yes - If free of cornstarch and corn syrup

Meats and Proteins:

Food	SCD	My Diet
Fresh meats (ex: chicken, pork, fish)	Yes	Yes
Processed Meats	No	No
Hot dogs	No	Yes - If free of starches
Bacon	Yes - If free of sugars	Yes - If free of corn syrup
Canned Tuna	Yes	Yes - If in water only
Eggs	Yes	Yes
Tofu	No	Yes
Tempeh	No	Yes - If free of barley
Nuts	Yes	Yes - If free of starches
Peanut Butter	Yes - If free of added sugars	Yes - If free of corn syrup
High Starch Beans (ex: soybeans, chickpeas, fava beans)	No	Yes - If free of sauces and corn syrup
Low Starch Beans (ex: white beans, lentils, lima beans)	Yes	Yes - If free of sauces and corn syrup
Split peas	Yes	Yes

Drinks:

Food	SCD	My Diet
Coffee	No	Yes - If sweetened with natural sugar
Tea (caffeinated, herbal)	Yes - If unsweetened	Yes - If sweetened with natural sugar
Soda	No	Yes - If sweetened with natural sugar
Diet Soda	Yes	No
Seltzer Water	Yes	Yes
Fruit Juices	Yes - If free of added sugars	Yes - If free of corn syrup
Coconut Milk	Yes	Yes
Coconut Water	No	Yes
Sweet Wine	No	Yes
Dry Wine	Yes	Yes
Beer	Yes	No
Gin	Yes	No
Scotch	Yes	No
Bourbon	Yes	No
Whiskey	Yes	No
Vodka	Yes	No
Brandy	No	Yes

Sugars:

Food	SCD	My Diet
White Sugar	No	Yes
Brown Sugar	No	Yes
Powdered Sugar	Yes - If free of corn starch	Yes - If free of corn starch
Honey	Yes	Yes
Corn Syrup	No	No
Agave Syrup	No	Yes
Maple Syrup	No	Yes - If free of corn syrup
Lactose	No	Yes
Fructose	No	No
Dextrose	No	No
Molasses	No	Yes
Date Sugar	No	Yes
Saccharine	Yes	No
Stevia	No	Yes
Splenda	No	No
Xylitol	No	No
Aspartame	No	No

Vinegars:

Food	SCD	My Diet
Distilled White Vinegar	Yes	No
White Wine Vinegar	Yes	Yes
Apple Cider Vinegar	Yes	Yes
Rice Vinegar	Yes	Yes
Balsamic Vinegar	No	Yes

Miscellaneous:

Food	SCD	My Diet
Carbs (ex: Pastas, breads, bagels)	No	No
Desserts (ex: Donuts, cookies, muffins, cakes)	No	No
Chocolate	No	Yes
Candy Licorice	No	No
Unflavored Gelatin	Yes	Yes
Flavored Gelatin	No	Yes

Miscellaneous (cont.):

Food	SCD	My Diet
Condiments (ex: ketchup, mustard, mayonnaise)	Yes - If free of added sugars	Yes - If free of corn syrup and white distilled vinegar
Soy Sauce	No	Yes - If Gluten Free
Kimchi	Yes	Yes
Most Oils (including sunflower, safflower, olive, canola, vegetable)	Yes	Yes - Except for corn oil
Soybean Oil	No	Yes
Spices	Yes	Yes - If free of starches
Baking Soda	Yes	Yes
Baking Powder	Yes - If free of corn starch	Yes - If free of corn starch
Chewing Gum	Yes - If made with saccharine	No
Guar Gum	No	Yes
Xanthan Gum	No	No
Lecithin	Yes	Yes

These two diets are fairly similar, though the SCD is much more restrictive. Generally speaking, the SCD does not allow for any starches or carbohydrates. My diet only excludes gluten containing grains such as wheat and barley, and corn derivatives. I can eat starchy vegetables, like potatoes, carrots and peas, rice, sugars, beans, and legumes. These are not allowed on the SCD.

My diet excludes distilled white vinegar and products that contain it. All other vinegars are ok to eat like apple cider, wine and balsamic. The SCD allows all vinegar except balsamic, which contains sugars, and sometimes natural apple cider vinegar.

Both diets exclude all foods that contain corn starch. This means even no baking powder or powdered sugar which both contain corn. The SCD also does not allow milk products. I can eat milk products, except for ones that contain vinegar, such as ricotta cheese.

As far as alcohol goes, I do not drink any that is made from grains, such as whiskey, vodka, scotch or beer. The SCD allows only for unsweetened drinks, so wine and brandy are excluded, but the other drinks are not.

Making Substitutions

It is harder than you would think to just eliminate foods or food groups from a diet. When possible it is always best to try and substitute. Fortunately we live in a time where all sorts of gluten free and allergen foods are available everywhere. Below are a few examples of substitutions that I make without feeling deprived.

Instead of this:	Use this:
White vinegar	Apple cider or balsamic vinegar
Mayonnaise	Vegenaise (made with apple cider vinegar)
Pancake syrup (full of high fructose corn syrup)	Pure maple syrup
Wheat Pasta	Delallo's (gluten free)
Couscous	Quinoa
Regular soda (high fructose corn syrup)	Pepsi - Real Sugar (made with real sugar only)

Instead of this:	Use this:
Soy sauce (full of gluten)	Kikkoman or Braggs Liquid Aminos (gluten free soy sauce or soy sauce substitute)
Baking powder (mixed with cornstarch)	Featherweight (corn free)
Sweetened yogurt	Oui (made with real sugar)
Tortillas	Siete (gluten and corn free)
Bagels	Against the Grain (gluten and corn free)
Frozen waffles	Van's (gluten and corn free)
Cereal	Chex gluten free, Van's, or Bob Mills Muesli (gluten and corn free)
Canned Tomato soup	Amy's Tomato soup
Macaroni and cheese	Amy's gluten free Macaroni and cheese
Granola bars	Van's (gluten and corn free)

Instead of this:	Use this:
Cookies	Glutino gluten free wafers, Tates gluten free cookies, or Betty Crocker gluten free cookie mix
Seasoned rice	Near East Long Grain rice

The most important thing I did was to become a label reader. I read the full list of ingredients each time I would buy something new. Sometimes I had to do a little detective work and research certain ingredients. Different brands have different ingredients and it's important not to assume that a certain brand is safe without double checking the ingredients. I understand that it's a little exhausting at first but once I found brands that worked, I would stick with them. I also read labels with each purchase since ingredients are subject to change.

Please feel free to visit my blog as I update and review new products:

https://howibeatcrohns-lynne.blogspot.com

The Good Years

You may be wondering how I can be confident that this diet has worked for me. How do I know that my disease didn't just go into remission on its own and had nothing to do with my diet? What proof do I have that my diet is linked to my remission? Could I have gone into remission at the same time that I was trying out this new diet?

A few years back I had a colonoscopy. Though I had several in the past before my new diet, this was the first one since going gluten and corn free. It was a little scary since I was still having flares once in a while when I accidentally ate something I shouldn't have. Well, after doing the colonoscopy I came back *negative* for Crohn's! There was no sign that I was suffering from Crohn's disease.

Ok, a little bit technical, but follow me here. Along with the colonoscopy I had had a few other tests done. I had a blood test done for high levels of c-reactive protein which turned out to be negative. A high level of c-reactive protein in the blood indicates that there is chronic and long term inflammation somewhere in the body. It does not specify a place in the body, so it can be caused by anything from Crohn's to cancer [30]. If my test had come back positive for high levels of c-reactive protein it could have indicated I had Crohn's. In fact, it should have been high for someone with active Crohn's. I also had a CT scan of the small intestines, which was negative as well. Both of these tests pick up on inflammation in the body. People with Crohn's will test high for c-reactive protein. People with Crohn's disease may show some inflammation on the CT scan. Here's where it gets interesting. About a week before my scheduled colonoscopy I had a stool sample tested for calprotectin, a protein which was significantly higher in my body than it should have been. This particular protein is known to be elevated when there is any inflammation specifically in the colon. Calprotectin will show inflammation that goes back up to a few weeks in the past. This can be from a major flare or from a little irritation from something such as a food or a virus [31,32,33].

Why was this Calprotectin test being elevated so interesting? Because my colon was inflamed from a mistake I had in my diet a few days earlier. Two days prior to the test, I had accidentally eaten fish in a restaurant that had cornstarch on it. I try to be careful, but still make mistakes once in a while. Usually fish is a fairly safe food for me to order in a restaurant. However, this one came with a nice pesto on top. Under the pesto I could see the white powder. I stopped eating at this point but had probably eaten about a third of the filet. Next day, bloody diarrhea! Lasted only one day. There was some short term irritation in my colon that was directly related to the fish. A few days later and my calprotectin level was elevated due to the short term inflammation. It makes sense that it would be elevated while my other tests were negative. My tests had shown that I had some recent inflammation, but not chronic, or long term.

Fast forward to the colonoscopy a couple weeks later. My doctor said that he was confused that the calprotectin could be elevated but everything else was negative. It didn't make sense to him that the long term markers didn't show any inflammation. He even told me that he had initially considered canceling the colonoscopy to give my body a chance to calm down from the inflammation. He expected there to be a lot of inflammation because of the elevated calprotectin. I told him about the fish incident. I explained how eating certain foods made me flare and that if I avoided these foods I was fine. I think he thought I was nuts! He went into the colonoscopy expecting to find inflammation, which he did not. He said that I did not have Crohn's right now! Well, I did, and it somehow had managed to go into complete remission. What is so important about this is that my remission occurred at the same time that I went back to my gluten free and corn free diet.

After that, the next few years were relatively good. Yes, I still had flares once in a while, but they were short lived. Once in a while I would make a mistake and I would get sick. This is something that I had to dedicate my whole life to doing. Every time I put something into my mouth, it was taking a risk. And if I did make a mistake, it could take days if not weeks for my colon to right itself again.

Grocery shopping was quite a chore and took a lot of time. I needed to read the ingredients on every label. I knew everything that was going into my mouth. If I didn't recognize an ingredient I would look it up to see if it was a possible derivative of wheat and corn. I started with products in the gluten free section and then made sure that they were also free from corn and corn derivatives.

I compared brands. Sometimes different brands have different ingredients. One brand may use high fructose corn syrup while another brand may use granulated sugar. And to complicate things even more, some products would change their ingredients for no apparent reason and without warning. So even if I had eaten a product safely for many months or years, I had to constantly check labels.

Eating out at restaurants was always a risk. I would try to ask the waiter general questions about the food, but it was never really enough to be completely sure I would be safe. Sometimes I took a gamble. If I flared the next day after going to a restaurant I knew to not order that food again. Likewise, through trial and error I also learned which foods I could order at different restaurants. This, of course, is assuming that they didn't change the ingredients between my visits. Let us say I don't eat out that often.

When I do eat out, I try to always stick with the safest options. That means no sauces or gravies on meat. No salad dressings. Fish is a relatively safe item, as long as it was just baked and not breaded. Cooked vegetables are generally good as long as they're not mixed with corn.

It also tended to be difficult when eating at a relative's or friend's house. I remember one particular time at my friend's mom's house. She was famous for her sweet and sour meatballs. I asked her if there was any wheat in it. She answered, "Oh no, no, just bread crumbs". This is just one example of many, where relatives are well meaning and care about you, but are not knowledgeable enough to know all the ingredients or sources of ingredients.

I still remember the first time I tried flying fish eggs. They are the tiny orange eggs they use in sushi and they are quite honestly delicious. When you buy them in an asian supermarket in a plastic container, there are no ingredients listed. I figured they were just eggs and nothing more. Well, I got really sick the next day. A quick search on the computer showed that they are soaked in soy sauce and corn syrup. No wonder they tasted so good. I will rarely buy foods that do not list ingredients.

Once in a while I would have a flare that I honestly have no idea why it happened. It usually followed a visit to a restaurant or a relatives' house where I didn't have full access to the all the ingredients. The flare would be super mild, usually just a drop of blood, and would pass quickly. But it was enough to let me know that I had eaten something wrong and that I needed to be more careful.

In general I have been feeling really good since making this discovery about myself. I work full time with children at a daycare center. This job requires an exceptional amount of energy. I cannot leave the room whenever I need to go to the bathroom. I'm also very active and love to exercise. I enjoy hiking, running, yoga, tennis, basketball and weight lifting. I feel generally pretty good all day. The best part is that I am not in the bathroom 20 times per day!

Another thing that I have been able to do is travel. Though the eating out can be a challenge at times, I have been able to steer free of most foods that would flare me by getting the safest options. I am able to sit for long car or plane rides and not worry. I can enjoy walking around somewhere all day and not worry about being close enough to a bathroom.

An additional thing I have learned to do is to always carry snacks with me. I call them my 'emergency foods'. These are snacks that are portable and don't need refrigerated, such as protein bars, almonds, or carrot sticks. They aren't meant to be meals, but are enough to hold me over until I can find some good food options. These have saved me from making bad decisions when I get hungry.

Dealing With Relatives

I am gluten and corn free. None of my other family members are gluten and corn free, though some of them have their own food allergies to watch. I do not want to unfairly subject them to my diet restrictions. This is my diet, not theirs. But they live with me and I want us to eat dinner together as a family. Some changes had to be made.

In my house I have lots of foods that are gluten free and also lots of foods that are not. I shop for both kinds of pastas. I boil two separate pots for the pasta, one for regular and one for the gluten free. I am used to the gluten free pasta, but it doesn't really compare to regular. When I do this I have to be extra careful not to mix them up, which can easily happen.

Some substitutions won't make any difference in tastes, like when using different brands. White distilled vinegar is often derived from corn. This is a big no-no for me. There are also some sour creams that contain vinegar and some that don't. There is really no difference between these brands as far as taste goes. So I just buy the one that does not use vinegar.

Sometimes there is just a difference in the method of preparation. I may prepare a breaded food for my family, and then just make the same thing for myself without the breading. I try hard not to deprive them of anything. It is my diet, not theirs.

I still buy things at the store that I cannot eat, including cookies, bread and crackers. They are for my family and I know not to go near them. I know that I have to stick to this diet one hundred percent, so I am actually not even tempted. But this means that I do have to practice 'mindful eating'. I need to be very aware of everything that I put in my mouth. I have to think about all of the ingredients. I also have to be sure if a food is mine or if it is meant for my family. Things can get mixed up pretty easily.

I always try to think ahead and plan meals before I get hungry. Once my sugar level drops I'm more likely to make a mistake. I'm also more likely to live life on the edge when I'm already hungry, taking chances on foods that I'm not really sure of. That is another reason that I like to carry snacks with me, especially if I plan to be out for a while shopping and doing errands.

Related Diseases

It is my theory that there are actually a lot of autoimmune diseases that are caused by, or exacerbated by food sensitivities. I believe this is true of Crohn's disease. But there are some other auto-autoimmune diseases that may also be managed through diet.

One of these diseases is Relapsing Polychondritis. I was diagnosed with this around the same time that I was diagnosed with Crohn's disease. It is characterized by inflammation of the cartilage in the body, including the bridge of the nose and the outer ear. These symptoms also went away when I eliminated the gluten and corn from my diet.

Another big one is eczema. My daughter had suffered from this as an infant and it was quite severe. We took countless trips to the doctor, looking for something that would help. We tried everything from certain soaps and lotions to changing our laundry detergent. Nothing seemed to work. Due to the eczema, she was not sleeping well and the doctor prescribed Benadryl liquid. Well, we tried it and it turned out to be the worst night of itching scratching she ever had. Looking at the label, the first ingredient other than the medicine itself was citric acid. Could this actually be causing her eczema? I took her off of all citric acid and made my own baby food instead of using store bought food (which almost always contains citric acid as a preservative). Her eczema started to clear up within days.

This same daughter suffered from neuropathy in her teenage

years. She had tingling sensations as well as numbness in her tongue. She also had weird sensations and pains. We went to a neurologist who did every test imaginable, and found nothing. As she had gotten older she had started to eat foods with citric acid in them again. In fact lately she had been drinking a whole lot of wassail juice, made with orange, lemon and pineapple juices. I wondered if this could be causing the problem. It took a few weeks off of citric acid, but the symptoms went away.

As amazing as all of this is, it is true. I also have noticed that people tend to have not one, but several autoimmune diseases at the same time, or disease clustering. I have Crohn's disease and also Relapsing Polychondritis. I feel that these are just different ways that the body reacts to foods that it is sensitive to. These food triggers can affect the digestive tract (Crohn's), the skin (Eczema), joints (Arthritis), cartilage (Relapsing Polychondritis), nervous system (Neuropathy), etc.

Recipes

On the following pages I have included some of my favorite recipes that are both gluten and corn free. They are also free of many other common allergens. I have also listed some recommended brands that I like to use in my recipes.

For additional recipes check out my blog:
www.HowIbeatCrohns-lynne.blogspot.com.

Breakfast

Berry Smoothie Bowl

Ingredients:

- 1 ½ cup milk (or milk substitute)
- ½ frozen banana
- ¼ cup fresh spinach
- 1 cup frozen mixed berries
- 1 or 2 tbs. protein powder

Suggested toppings:
- ½ fresh banana, (sliced)
- ½ cup fresh berries
- ¼ cup granola (gluten and corn free)
- 1 tbs. chocolate chips
- 1 tbs. honey

Directions:

1. Add the milk, banana, spinach, berries, and protein powder to a blender.
2. Blend mixture until smooth.
3. Pour into a bowl and top with desired toppings such as fresh banana, berries, granola, chocolate chips, and honey.

Makes 2 servings

Suggestions:

- I like to use Warrior brand powdered protein which is gluten and corn free.
- Try customizing your bowl by adding your favorite toppings. I like to sometimes add other healthy toppings like coconut, almonds, and chia seeds.

Chocolate Holiday Crepes

Ingredients:

- 1 cup flour
- 1 tbs. sugar
- 3 eggs
- 1 1/4 cup milk (or milk substitute

- 3 tbs. melted butter
- 1/4 cup powdered sugar (cornstarch free)
- 4 tbs. Nutella

Directions:

1. Mix together flour and sugar; set aside.
2. In a large bowl, beat eggs, and milk together.
3. Gradually beat in flour mixture until smooth.
4. Melt butter in a pan over medium-high heat. Pour batter onto pan with around 2 tbs. batter for each crepe.
5. Swirl batter to evenly coat pan.
6. Cook for about 1 minute or until lightly browned; gently flip using a spatula or tongs. Cook for another 30 seconds or until browned and remove from pan.
7. Spread Nutella and roll the crepe. Top with more Nutella and powdered sugar.

Makes 8 crepes.

Suggestions:

- I like to use Wholesome brand organic powdered sugar which is free of cornstarch.
- Try adding fresh fruit and bacon for a delicious holiday treat.

Oatmeal Bars To-Go

Ingredients:

- 1 banana
- 1 egg
- 1 1/4 milk (or milk substitute)
- 1/2 cup applesauce
- 1 tsp. vanilla extract
- 1/3 cup brown sugar
- 1/4 tsp. salt
- 2 1/2 cups gluten free oats
- 2 tbs. flaxseed meal
- 1/2 tsp. cinnamon
- 1/2 cup chocolate chips

Directions:

1. Preheat oven to 350 °F.
2. In a large bowl, mix together banana, egg, milk, applesauce, vanilla and sugar and salt.
3. Mix in oats, flaxseed, and cinnamon.
4. Fold in chocolate chips.
5. Butter a casserole dish and pour in oatmeal mix.
6. Bake for 35 to 40 minutes.
7. Cut into squares and serve.

Makes about 16 servings.

Suggestions:

- Try adding other healthy ingredients like unsalted nuts or dried fruit.

Banana Chocolate Chip Pancakes

Ingredients:

- 2 eggs
- 1 ripe banana
- 1/4 cup milk (or milk substitute)
- 1 tsp. vanilla extract
- 1/3 cup oat flour
- 1/3 cup rice flour
- 1/3 cup almond flour
- 1 tbs. ground flaxseed
- 1/2 tsp. baking soda
- 1/2 tsp. of cinnamon
- 1/4 tsp. of salt
- 1/2 cup chocolate chips
- 2 tbs. butter

Directions:

1. Add eggs, banana, milk, and vanilla to a blender.
2. Blend mixture until smooth.
3. Add in remaining dry ingredients (except for the chocolate chips); blend until smooth.
4. Fold in chocolate chips.
5. Melt butter in a pan over medium heat.
6. Pour in batter.
7. Allow pancake to cook until golden brown on each side.
8. Remove from pan and serve with maple syrup if desired.

Makes about 12 small pancakes.

Suggestions:

- Always be sure to use pure maple syrup. Other commercial brands tend to add corn syrup.
- A great egg substitute to try is flaxseed:
    1 egg = 1 tbs. flaxseed and 3 tbs. water
    Mix and let sit for 5 minutes to thicken.

Fried Potatoes with Green Peppers and Kale

Ingredients:

- 3 large potatoes
- 5 large kale leaves
- 1 green pepper
- 2 tbs. olive oil
- salt and pepper (to taste)

Directions:

1. Cut pepper into bite sized pieces; thoroughly wash kale leaves and tear off pieces while leaving central stem behind.
2. Cut potatoes into slices.
3. In a large skillet, heat oil over medium-high heat.
4. Add potatoes to the pan and cook for about 5 minutes.
5. Add green pepper; cook for about 10 minutes and stirring occasionally.
6. Add in kale until cooked down and potatoes are soft and golden brown (about 5 minutes).
7. Season with salt and pepper to taste.

Makes 4 servings.

Please note: Potatoes are restricted if following the Specific Carbohydrate Diet; although I have never had a problem with them.

Suggestions:

- Try throwing in other healthy veggies like broccoli, onion, or sweet bell peppers.

Apple Donuts

Ingredients:

- 2 apples
- 4 tbs. peanut butter (or other nut butter)
- 2 tsp. raisins
- 2 tsp. ground flaxseed
- 2 tsp. gluten free oats
- 2 tsp. chia seeds

Directions:

1. Cut the top and bottom off of each apple and discard.
2. Cut the apple into 1/2 inch slices; carve out the center core; dry the top of each apple slice.
3. Spread the peanut butter (other nut butter; almond is especially good) evenly over each apple slice.
4. Top with raisins, flaxseed, oats, and chia seeds.
5. Enjoy this yummy and healthy breakfast treat!

Makes 2 servings.

Suggestions:

- I love this recipe because you can get really creative! Try different spreads like Nutella or flavored yogurt. I also love adding toppings like berries, nuts, or chocolate chips.
- Make sure to dry each apple before you add a spreads to help stick better to the surface of the apple.

Eggs with Dinosaur Kale

Ingredients:

- 4 eggs
- 1 tbs. milk (or milk substitute)
- 6 dinosaur kale leaves
- 1 tbs. butter
- salt and pepper (to taste)

Directions:

1. Thoroughly wash kale leaves and strip them from the stems.
2. Chop the kale leaves into smaller 1-2 inch pieces.
3. Melt butter in a pan over medium heat. Add kale and cook for 3-5 minutes until kale wilts down; stirring occasionally.
4. Crack eggs into a small bowl. Add milk with a dash of salt and whisk.
5. Pour into the pan and allow the eggs to thoroughly coat the kale.
6. Stir until eggs are fully cooked.
7. Add salt and pepper to taste and enjoy!

Makes 2 servings.

Suggestions:

- What's scrambled eggs without cheese? Try adding mozzarella or cheddar cheese just before the eggs are fully cooked for a delicious cheesy extra.

Main Dishes

Lentil Cabbage Soup (Vegan)

Ingredients:

- 2 potatoes
- 3/4 head of cabbage
- 1/2 yellow onion
- 4 carrots
- 5 garlic cloves
- 1/4 cup dry lentils
- 8 cups water

- 1 cup frozen spinach
- 1 can tomato sauce (10 oz)
- 1 tbs. miso paste
- 1 tbs. soy sauce (gluten free)
- 1 tbs. curry
- 1 tbs. brown sugar
- 1 tbs. olive oil

Directions:

1. Peel and dice potatoes into bite sized pieces.
2. Lightly chop cabbage and onion; slice up carrots; mince garlic.
3. Rinse off lentils.
4. Fill a large pot with water; add all ingredients.
5. Bring pot to a boil; simmer covered over medium heat for around 2 hours and stir occasionally.

Makes 6 servings.

Suggestions:

- Kikkoman makes a great version of gluten free soy sauce. I also like to sometimes use Bragg's amino acids as a great soy-free soy sauce substitute.

Rice and Lentils

Ingredients:

- 1 cup dry rice
- 1/3 cup dry lentils
- 1/3 cup split peas
- 1 tbs. olive oil
- 1/2 tsp. turmeric
- salt (to taste)
- 1/2 cup fresh parsley (chopped)

Directions:

1. Cook rice (either in a rice steamer or on the stove).
2. Fill a large pot with water and bring to a boil.
3. Add lentils and split peas to the pot; boil for 25 minutes and stir occasionally.
4. Drain the lentils and peas. Return to pot and stir in the cooked rice.
5. Season individual servings with olive oil, turmeric and salt to taste.
6. Top with parsley.

Makes 6 servings.

Suggestions:

- This is a great staple food I love to eat all the time. Try mixing it up by tossing in some roasted veggies and egg.

Stir-Fry Chicken with Quinoa

Ingredients:

- 1 pound chicken breast
- 1 medium zucchini
- 1 red pepper
- 2 cups broccoli
- 2 green onions
- 3 cups quinoa (when cooked)

- 2 tbs. olive oil
- 1/2 tsp. curry
- 1/2 tsp. garlic powder
- 1 tsp. honey
- 2 tsp. soy sauce (gluten free)
- 1/2 tsp. salt
- red pepper flakes (to taste)

Directions:

1. Dice red pepper, zucchini, and broccoli; chop up green onion.
2. Cut up the chicken into smaller bite sized pieces; pat dry with paper towels.
3. In a small bowl combine garlic powder, honey, 1 tsp. soy sauce, salt, curry, and red pepper flakes.
4. Add olive oil to a pan on medium-high heat; add chicken.
5. Add the sauce to the chicken and toss to coat; cook until chicken is lightly browned and cooked through.
6. Add olive oil to a separate pan on medium heat; add in vegetables and remaining soy sauce. Cook until vegetables are tender.
7. Serve chicken and vegetables over quinoa and enjoy.

Makes 4 servings.

Suggestions:

- If you aren't a fan of quinoa, try rice instead which makes this meal just as good.
- Get creative with your veggies and toss in whatever you like. I sometimes like to add greens or mushrooms.

Tuna Noodle Casserole

Ingredients:

- 1 package of gluten free curly pasta (12 oz)
- 1 tbs. butter
- 2 cans tuna (12 oz each)
- 2 cans creamy mushroom soup (14 oz each)
- 1/4 cup milk (or milk substitute)
- 1 cup frozen spinach (thawed)
- 1/2 cup shredded cheddar cheese
- 1/2 cup potato chips (crumbled)

Directions:

1. Preheat oven to 350 °F.
2. Bring a large pot of water to a boil and cook pasta according to package directions.
3. In a large bowl, combine pasta, tuna, mushroom soup, milk, spinach and cheese; mix well.
4. Butter a casserole dish; pour in the mix.
5. Sprinkle the top with extra cheese; bake casserole for 40 minutes.
6. Crumble up chips and sprinkle onto the casserole; bake another 5 minutes. Serve and enjoy!

Makes 10 servings.

Suggestions:

- I like to use Amy's Porcini mushroom soup for this recipe.
- Make sure that you tuna is packaged in water. Sometimes the oil packaged tuna contains corn, so be careful and read the ingredients.
- Always be careful about chips as well since a lot of them are make with corn. I like to use original Cape Cod chips which are a safe brand with no corn added.

Pan-Yang Chicken Curry

Ingredients:

- 1 1/2 cups dry rice
- 2 potatoes
- 4 carrots
- boneless skinless chicken (12 oz package)
- 2 tbs. olive oil
- 1 head of broccoli
- 2 tsp. ginger
- 2 tbs. soy sauce (gluten free)
- 5 garlic cloves (minced)
- 1/4 cup peanut butter (or other nut butter)
- 1 can coconut milk (13.5 oz)
- 1 tsp. turmeric
- 1 tsp. cumin
- 1 tsp. chili powder
- 4 tsp. curry powder
- 2 tbs. gluten free flour

Directions:

1. Cook rice according to packaged directions.
2. Dice potato and carrots into bite sized pieces; boil in water until tender (make sure to save 3 cups of the water for later).
3. Heat 1 tbs. olive oil over medium heat; cook broccoli until tender.
4. Cut chicken into bite sized pieces; pay dry.
5. Heat remaining olive oil over medium-high heat; cook chicken until browned and cooked through.
6. Add reserved water to a large pot; mix in all remaining ingredients.
7. Mix in chicken and vegetables. Serve over rice and enjoy.

Makes 8 servings.

Suggestions:

- If you're not a fan of chicken try adding a different protein like tofu.

Quinoa Bowl with Vegetables and Walnuts

Ingredients:

- 1 1/2 cup dry quinoa
- 1 large yellow onion
- 1 bunch of asparagus
- 2 zucchinis
- 1/2 head of broccoli
- 5 garlic cloves

- 3 tbs. olive oil
- 1/2 cup parmesan cheese
- 1/2 cup walnuts
- 1 lemon
- salt and pepper (to taste)

Directions:

1. Preheat oven to 450 °F; prepare quinoa according to package.
2. Chop asparagus stalks and broccoli into bite sized pieces; slice zucchini in thin circles; mince garlic; dice onion;
3. Toss asparagus, broccoli, and zucchini with 2 tbs. olive oil; add salt and pepper to taste. Roast vegetables on a baking sheet until lightly browned (15-20 minutes).
4. Heat remaining olive oil in a pan over medium-high heat. Toss in onion and cook until soft (about 4 minutes); add garlic and cook 1 minute more.
5. Toss onion and garlic into the pot with cooks quinoa; stir in juice from 1/2 lemon, 2 tbsp. butter, and 1/4 cup of cheese.
6. Divide quinoa and serve with vegetables; top with walnuts and the remaining cheese.

Makes 4 servings.

Suggestions:

- If you aren't a fan of quinoa, try rice instead. It can be just as tasty.

Beef Bibimbap with Vegetables

Ingredients:

- 2 zucchini
- 1 package of button mush-rooms (8 oz)
- 4 green scallions
- 4 carrots
- 2 tbs. fresh ginger
- 5 garlic cloves
- salt and pepper (to taste)

- 1 1/2 cups dry rice
- 2 tbs. sesame oil
- 3 tbs. sugar
- 4 tsp. sriracha
- 6 tbs. soy sauce
- 8 tsp. olive oil
- ground beef (20 oz)

Directions:

1. Thinly slice zucchini, mushrooms, and scallions. Use a peeler to shave carrots into long ribbons. Mince garlic and ginger.
2. Prepare rice according to package directions.
3. In a large pan heat 2 tsp. olive oil over medium-high heat. Cook carrots until tender and season with salt and pepper; remove from pan. Repeat step 3 with zucchini and then with the mushrooms.
4. Heat remaining olive oil in a pan over medium-high heat; add ginger and garlic and cook for 1 minute. Add beef and cook until no longer pink; over high heat cook until meat is browned and crisp.
5. Add 3 tbsp. soy sauce; cook for another 2 minutes.
6. In a small bowl mix together sesame oil, sugar, 2 tsp. sriracha, and remaining soy sauce.
7. Divide rice and top with the beef and vegetables. Add sauce, remaining sriracha (to taste), and garnish with scallions.

Makes 4 servings.

Easy Pad Thai

Ingredients:

- 1 package gluten free noodles (curly or penne) (12 oz)
- 1/2 head of cauliflower
- 1 1/2 cup spinach
- 1 green onion
- 3 tbs. olive oil
- 1/2 container tofu (extra firm) (pressed)
- 1/2 cup butter
- 3/4 cup peanut butter (or other nut butter)
- 1 tbsp. soy sauce
- 2 tbs. brown sugar
- red pepper flakes (to taste)
- 1 leftover chicken breast, shredded (optional)

Directions:

1. Prepare noodles according to package directions
2. Chop cauliflower; thinly slice green onion; cube tofu.
3. Heat 1 tbs. olive oil in pan over medium heat. Cook cauliflower until soft; add spinach and green onion; cook until spinach softens.
4. In another pan over medium heat, prepare sauce by mixing butters, remaining olive oil, soy sauce, brown sugar, and pepper flakes.
5. Add noodles, tofu, vegetables, and chicken (optional) to sauce. Stir to coat and enjoy.

Makes 4 servings.

Suggestions:

- Try adding different veggies. Broccoli and mung bean sprouts go great with this recipe.

Pasta with Veal in Marsala Sauce

Ingredients:

- 1 package gluten free spaghetti noodles (12 oz)
- 1 lb. ground veal
- Portabella mushrooms (8 oz package), washed and sliced
- 2 tbs. olive oil
- 2 tbs. butter
- 1 cup milk (or milk substitute)
- 1/2 cup marsala wine
- 2 cups chicken stock
- 3 shallots, chopped
- 1 celery stalk, chopped
- 2 tbs. tomato paste
- 4 cloves garlic, minced
- 1/8 tsp. nutmeg
- salt and pepper (to taste)
- 2 tbs. fresh thyme, chopped
- 1 tbs. fresh sage, chopped

Directions:

1. Cook noodles according to package directions.
2. In a large skillet over medium-high heat, add olive oil. Add veal, mushrooms, butter, nutmeg, salt, and pepper. Cook until veal is browned.
3. Add shallots, celery, garlic, thyme, and sage. Cook for 4-5 minutes.
4. Stir in tomato paste. Simmer for 4-5 minutes.
5. Add milk, wine, and chicken stock. Simmer for 30 minutes.
6. Pour sauce over pasta and enjoy.

Makes 5 servings.

Suggestions:

- Absolutely delicious recipe and makes gluten free noodles really tasty!
- Try sprinkling in some parmesan cheese for an even tastier dish.

Side Dishes

Cauliflower with Paprika and Butter

Ingredients:

- 1 head cauliflower
- 4 creen onions, sliced
- 4 tbs. butter
- 1 tbs. paprika

Directions:

1. Wash and cut cauliflower into small, bite sized pieces.
2. Place cauliflower in a microwaveable dish with 1/2 cup water.
3. Cover with a paper towel; steam until tender (about 9 minutes, stirring halfway through).
4. In a pan over medium heat, saute onions in butter then add paprika.
5. Drain any water remaining from cauliflower dish.
6. Add butter sauce to cauliflower and stir to coat.

Makes 4 servings.

Homemade Applesauce

Ingredients:

- 8 - 10 apples (variety)
- 1/2 cup water
- 1/2 cup sugar
- 1 tsp. cinnamon

Directions:

1. Peel, core, and dice apples into pieces.
2. Place all ingredients into a crockpot.
3. Cook on high until apples are soft (about 4 hours).
4. Mash with a potato masher until at desired consistency.

Makes 4 servings.

Suggestions:

- It's best to try using a variety of apples. I usually like to throw in a few green apples to the mix for a more tart taste.

Chilean Celery Avocado Salad

Ingredients:

- 2 avocados, peeled, deseeded, and cubed
- 1 head of celery
- 1 lemon
- 2 tbsp. olive oil
- salt and pepper (to taste)

Directions:

1. Wash celery and dice into small pieces.
2. Mix in avocados.
3. Juice the lemon and add to the salad; drizzle with olive oil.
4. Add salt and pepper to taste.
5. Mix well and enjoy.

Makes 4 servings.

Tabouli Salad with Quinoa

Ingredients:

- 1 cup quinoa
- 1 bunch fresh parsley
- 1 large tomato, diced
- 1/2 cucumber, diced
- 2 scallions, sliced
- 1 lemon
- 2 tbsp. olive oil
- salt and pepper (to taste)

Directions:

1. Bring 1 cup of water to a boil.
2. Add quinoa and cook according to package directions.
3. Roughly cut up parsley.
4. When quinoa is fully cooked, allow to cool to room temperature.
5. Add tomato, cucumber, and scallions.
6. Juice lemon and add to salad; drizzle salad with olive oil.
7. Add salt and pepper to taste; top with fresh parsley.

Makes 4 servings.

Suggestions:

- If you aren't a fan of quinoa, try rice instead. It can be just as tasty.

Corn Free and Gluten Free Bread

Ingredients:

- 3 eggs
- 3/4 cup milk (or milk substitute)
- 3 tbs. olive oil
- 1 tsp. honey
- 1 tbs. apple cider vinegar
- 1 1/2 tbs. yeast
- 1/2 tsp. baking powder
- 2 tbs. ground flaxseed
- 1 1/2 cup rice flour
- 1/2 cup gluten free oats
- 1/4 tsp. salt

Directions:

1. Preheat oven to 350 °F.
2. Combine all wet ingredients into a large bowl; mix well.
3. In a separate bowl, combine all dry ingredients; mix well.
4. Slowly stir in dry mixture into bowl with wet ingredients.
5. Coat bread pan with oil and add bread mixture to the pan.
6. Top with extra oats.
7. Bake for 45 to 50 minutes.

Makes 1 loaf bread

Notes:
- Featherweight baking powder does not contain cornstarch like other baking powders do.
- Bob's Mills makes gluten free oats.

Suggestions:
- This bread is absolutely delicious! I like to eat mine with butter or peanut butter on top.

Desserts

Chocolate Chip Banana Bread

Ingredients:

- 2 ripe bananas
- 2 eggs, beaten
- 1/2 cup milk (or milk substitute)
- 1 tsp. vanilla
- 1/2 cup applesauce
- 3/4 cup brown sugar
- 1/4 cup ground flaxseed
- 1/4 cup almond flour
- 1/2 cup gluten free oats
- 1 cup rice flour
- 2 tsp. baking powder
- 1/2 tsp. salt
- cinnamon (to taste)
- 1/2 cup chocolate chips

Directions:

1. Preheat oven to 350 °F.
2. Mash bananas in a large bowl.
3. Add all wet ingredients as well as sugar; mix well.
4. In a separate bowl, mix together dry ingredients in a separate bowl.
5. Slowly stir in dry mixture to bowl with wet ingredients.
6. Mix in chocolate chips.
7. Coat a bread pan with oil; add bread mixture to the pan.
8. Bake in oven for around 45 minutes.

Makes 1 loaf

Suggestions:

- Try playing around with different flours to try out different consistencies. I like to sometimes use 1/2 cup almond flour and 1/2 cup of rice flour.

Chocolate Avocado Pudding

Ingredients:

- 2 avocados, peeled, deseeded, and cubed
- 1/3 cup milk (or milk substitute)
- 2 tsp. vanilla extract
- 1/2 cup unsweetened cocoa powder
- 1/2 cup brown sugar
- 1 large pinch cinnamon (optional)

Directions:

1. Place all ingredients in a blender or food processor; blend until smooth.
2. Place pudding into a bowl and chill in refrigerator for 30 minutes.
3. Serve and enjoy!

Makes 4 servings

Notes:

- I love this recipe because the avocado adds a nice creaminess without saturated fats. Plus, it makes the pudding absolutely delicious!

Avocado and Black Bean Brownies

Ingredients:

- 1 tbs. flaxseed meal
- 1 can black beans (no salt) (15 oz.), drained and rinsed
- 1/2 cup sugar
- 1 avocado, peeled, deseeded, and cubed
- 3 tsp. coconut oil
- 1/4 tsp. baking soda
- 1/4 tsp. baking powder
- 2/3 cup cocoa powder
- 1/3 cup chocolate chips

Directions:

1. Preheat oven to 350 °F.
2. In a small bowl combine flaxseed and 2 1/2 tbsp. water; Stir well and set aside for 5 minutes to thicken.
3. In a blender, or food processor, add black beans, sugar, avocado, 2 tsp. coconut oil, and the flaxseed mixture. Blend until smooth.
4. Add in baking soda, baking powder, and cocoa powder. Blend again until smooth.
5. Add chocolate chips and fold into mixture.
6. Grease a baking dish with 1 tsp. coconut oil.
7. Pour mixture into the baking dish; bake 25-30 minutes.
8. Allow to cool before serving.

Notes:

- Make sure to use a corn free baking powder for this recipe, like Featherweight.

Flourless Chocolate Chip Cookies

Ingredients:

- 1 cup peanut butter (or other nut butter)
- 1 cup sugar
- 1 egg
- 1 tsp. baking powder
- chocolate chips (to taste)

Directions:

1. Preheat oven to 350 °F.
2. In a medium bowl mix all ingredients, except chocolate chips, until smooth.
3. Fold in chocolate chips.
4. On a greased baking sheet, place dollops of cookie dough spaced about 1 inch apart.
5. Bake for 12-15 minutes.

Additional Thoughts

One important thing to note is that Crohn's can flare up for many reasons, not just diet. Though diet may be able to control this disease for the most part, other factors such as illness, bad diarrhea, extreme stress and medication changes may also cause a flare. Whenever the body is stressed it is possible to see a flare.

I underwent surgery three years ago to have my thyroid removed. Despite my diet, the stress from the anesthesia, antibiotics, and physical strain on my body was enough to send me into a flare. However, I also underwent a separate surgery more recently. For one reason or another, I did not flare. There are so many factors besides diet that are involved and situations can change.

A change in medication can also set off a flare. In my own personal experience this has, unfortunately, happened many times. Two years ago I had my thyroid removed and was put on a thyroid replacement medication - Tirosint. In general, the medication itself didn't cause me any problems. But after a checkup with my doctor, it was decided that the Tirosint dosage should be lowered. Two days after a lower dose I began to flare. Working with my doctor, I finally found a dosage that didn't give me a flare.

The most important point that I want to make is that eliminating wheat, gluten, and corn from my diet worked for me personally. But I realize that everyone is different and the diet that works for me may or may not work for others. There are other food sensitivities out there that may trigger a flare in one person, while having no effect in someone else. Soy, eggs, fish, dairy, and many more food sensitivities may be what affects other people. This is why keeping a food diary is such a necessity.

I want to make another very important note: I would never recommend treating this disease without a doctor's care. Throughout the many years it took me after my Crohn's diagnoses to get to where I am today, I was always working with my doctors for guidance and following their recommendations. It is possible to have a doctor eventually eliminate medication if a diet proves to be effective, but only if a doctor believes that it is safe to do so. Never go off of any medications without discussing the decision with a doctor.

Beating Crohn's disease is not quick or easy. Although I learned what triggered my flares, it took me years to modify a diet that worked. Even now I sometimes find myself making mistakes that set me back again. But looking back on it, it was well worth it to take the path that I did. By deciding to change my diet, I no longer suffer from Crohn's disease. By taking control of my diet, I took my life back and beat Crohn's.

I am always available to answer any questions:

E-mail: lynne1408@earthlink.net
Blog: https://howibeatcrohns-lynne.blogspot.com
PO Box: P.O. Box 104
    Crescent, PA 15046-0104

Many blessings for a healthy life!

References

1,2   CrohnsandColitis.com staff, "Understanding Crohn's Disease". Crohns and Colitis, AbbVie (2016), www.crohnsandcolitis.com/crohns

3,9   Nordquist, Christian, "What is Crohn's Disease?". Medical News Today, Healthline Media (Jan 2019), www.medicalnewstoday.com/articles/151620.php

4   Crohn's And Colitis Foundation Staff, "Types of Crohn's Disease and Associated Symptoms". Crohn's and Colitis Foundation (2019), www.crohnscolitisfoundation.org/what-are-crohns-and-colitis/what-is-crohns-disease/types-of-crohns-disease.html

5   Schoenfeld, Adam MD and Wu, George Y., Md, PhD, "Crohn's Disease Symptoms, Causes, Diet, Treatment, and Life Expectancy". Medicine Net, Web MD, LLC (2019), www.medicinenet.com/crohns_disease/article.htm

6   NYU Langone Health Staff, "Diagnosing Inflammatory Bowel Disease in Adults". NYU Langone Health, NYU Langone Hospitals (2019), www.conditions/inflammatory-bowel-disease-in-adults/diagnosis

7   HealthEngine.com Staff (June 2006), "Wireless Capsule Enteroscopy (Capsule Endoscopy; Pill Cam). Health Engine, Health Engine (2019), www.au/info/wireless-capsule-enteroscopy-capsule-endoscopy-pill-cam

8,12   Mayo Clinic Staff, "Crohn's Disease". Mayo Clinic, Mayo Foundation For Medical Education and Research (2019), www.mayoclinic.org/diseases-conditions/crohns-disease/symptoms-causes/syc-20353304

10   CDC Staff, "Epidemiology of the IBD". CDC, Center For Disease Control and Prevention, U.S. Department of Health and Human Services (March 2015), www.cdc.gov/ibd/IBD-epidemiology.htm

11   Gastrointestinal Society Staff, "The Effects of Smoking on IBD". GI Society, Canadian Society of Intestinal Research, Gastrointestinal Society (2018), www.badgut.org/information-centre/a-z-digestive-topics/effects-smoking-ibd/

13   Freeman, Hugh J.(Mach 2008), "Colorectal Cancer Risk in Crohn's Disease".
World Journal of Gastroenterology, National Center For Biotechnology Information,
www.ncbi.nlm.nih.gov/pmc/articles/PMC2700422/

14   Web MD Staff, "Vitamins For Crohn's Disease". Web MD, Web MD LLC
(2019), www.webmd.com/ibd-crohns-disease/crohns-disease/crohns-vitamins#2

15,16   Crohn's and Colitis Staff, "Crohn's Treatments". Crohn's and Colitis, AbbVie
(2016), www.crohnsandcolitis.com/crohns/disease-treatment

17   Nall, Rachel, RN, MSN (October 2018), "Crohn's disease surgery: What to
know". Medical News Today, Healthline Media UK Ltdhttp, www.medicalnewsto-
day.com/articles/323236.php

18   Tresca, Amber J. (March 2019), "Facial Swelling Caused by Prednisone". Very
Well Health. About, Inc. (2019), www.verywellhealth.com/prednisone-facial-moon-
ing-1942983

19,20,22   Cleveland Clinic Staff, "Food Problems: Is it an Allergy or Intolerance".
Cleveland Clinic, Cleveland Clinic (2019), www.my.clevelandclinic.org/health/
diseases/10009-food-problems-is-it-an-allergy-or-intolerance

21   Web MD Staff, (October 2018), "Food Allergy or Something Else?", Web Md.
Web MD LLC (2005-2019), www.webmd.com/allergies/foods-allergy-intolerance#1

23,24   Celiac Disease Foundation Staff, "Sources of Gluten". Celiac Disease Foundation, Celiac Disease Foundation (1998-2019). www.celiac.org/gluten-free-living/
what-is-gluten/sources-of-gluten/

25   Rosen, Sharon, (April 2010), "Ingredients Derived From Corn-what to Avoid".
Live Corn Free, Blogger. www.livecornfree.com/2010/04/ingredients-derived-from-
corn-what-to.html

26   Silverman, Francie MSN, (February 2017), "corn Allergy Food List". Leaves of
Life, leaves of Life (2017). www.leavesoflife.com/corn-allergy-food-list/

27   Indorato, Debra A.,RD, LDN, (March 2015), "Milk Allergy Avoidance List". Kidswithfoodallergies.org (2014). www.kidswithfoodallergies.org/media/Milk-Allergy-Avoidance-List-Hidden-Names.pdf

28   Indorato, Debra A., RD, LDN, (March 2015), "Soy Allergy Avoidance List". Kids With Food Allergies, A division of the Asthma and Allergy Foundation (2015) www.kidswithfoodallergies.org/media/Soy-Allergy-Avoidance-List-Hidden-Names.pdf

29   Raman, Ryan, MS, RD, (July 2017), ""How to do an Elimination Diet and Why". Healthline, Healthline Media (2005-2019). www.healthline.com/nutrition/elimination-diet#section8

30   Schaeffer, Katie, Senior Editor, (December 2018), "C-Reactive Protein (CRP)". Lab tests online, American Association for Clinical Chemistry (AACC). www.labtestsonline.org/tests/c-reactive-protein-crp

31   Schaeffer, Katie, Senior Editor, (December 2018), "Calprotectin". Lab Tests online, American Association for Clinical Chemistry (AACC). www.labtestsonline.org/tests/calprotectin

32   G.I. Society Staff, (2015), "Fecal Calprotectin Test". G.I. Society, Gastrointestinal Society (2018). https://www.badgut.org/information-centre/a-z-digestive-topics/fecal-calprotectin-test/

33   Tresca, Amber J., (March 2019), "How The Fecal Calprotectin Test is Used in IBD". Very Well Health, About, Inc. (2019). https://www.verywellhealth.com/how-the-fecal-calprotectin-test-is-used-in-ibd-4140079

34   Harris, Cheryl, MPH, RD, (June 2017), Specific Carbohydrate Diet for Inflammatory Bowel Disease - Learn About the SCD to Support Clients With IBD and How it compares with other Evidence Based Natural Therapies". Today's Dietician, Great Valley Publishing Company, Inc. (2019). www.todaysdietitian.com/newarchives/0617p42.shtml

35   Seattle Hospital Press Release, (December 2016), Novel Diet Shows Promise in Treating Children with Crohn's Disease and Ulcerative Colitis". Seattle Children's Hospital. www.todaysdietitian.com/newarchives/0617p42.shtml